Priscila Piassi Carboni
Patrícia M. Pereira
Isabel C. Figueiredo

Speech therapy and orthognathic surgery

Priscila Piassi Carboni
Patrícia M. Pereira
Isabel C. Figueiredo

Speech therapy and orthognathic surgery

Orofacial myofunctional profile of patients undergoing orthognathic surgery

ScienciaScripts

Imprint

Cover image: www.ingimage.com

This book is a translation from the original published under ISBN 978-620-2-40429-7.

Publisher:
Sciencia Scripts
is a trademark of
Dodo Books Indian Ocean Ltd. and OmniScriptum S.R.L publishing group

120 High Road, East Finchley, London, N2 9ED, United Kingdom
Str. Armeneasca 28/1, office 1, Chisinau MD-2012, Republic of Moldova, Europe
Managing Directors: Ieva Konstantinova, Victoria Ursu
info@omniscriptum.com

Printed at: see last page
ISBN: 978-620-3-90129-0

DEDICATORY

To **God,** for the graces I have received throughout my life, which have been essential for me **to be where I am today.**

for me to be where I am today, and for allowing me to be part of the paths I have travelled

allowed me to be part of the paths I have travelled, in which I have acquired

knowledge and experiences that I will carry with me throughout my life.

To my mum, **Dulce**, for supporting me and dedicating herself to me every day, proving to me that she is a fighter and that with God by our side we can do anything, and that we can always overcome our limits.

To my siblings, **Sabrina** and **Frank**, for always supporting me and being for me when I needed them, even if they were far away.

ACKNOWLEDGEMENTS

To **God**, for always being by my side, enabling and blessing me in every
blessing me with every daily struggle and every challenge overcome. Giving me
strength in difficult times, and showing me how strong and capable I am
capable of achieving more and more. As well as putting marvellous wonderful people on my path this past year, who have helped me to remain steadfast in my goals until the end.

To **Fga. Isabel Cristina Figueiredo,** for her support, guidance and generosity.
generosity.
To **Fr**. **Patrícia**, for giving me the opportunity to continue her research.

To the **participants in** this study, who kindly made themselves available for the realisation of this work.

To my friends and **Fgas**. **Lia, Mariana, Jessica, Marinna, Isabella, Isabela** and **Bárbara**, for their daily support, advice, patience, companionship and, above all, for the friendship they provided this year.

To the **staff of the Outpatient Centre and Hospital de Base,** who contributed not only to my professional knowledge, but also to my personal knowledge.

EPIGRAPH

"Everything has its appointed time, and there is a time for every purpose under heaven".

Ecclesiastes 3:1

SUMMARY

CARBONI, P.P. Orofacial myofunctional profile of patients undergoing orthognathic surgery. [Monograph] São José do Rio Preto: São José do Rio Preto Medical School, 2014.

INTRODUCTION:

The stomatognathic system identifies a set of oral structures that perform common functions, with the mandible being a constant feature. Changes in the dynamics of this system interfere with craniofacial growth in such a way as to impair breathing, chewing, swallowing and speech. Orthodontic treatment combined with orthognathic surgery brings solutions to patients. Speech therapists are the professionals trained to carry out orofacial myofunctional therapy to restore stomatognathic functions and their balance. **OBJECTIVE**: To define orofacial myofunctional aspects in patients undergoing orthognathic surgery and post-operative speech therapy. **METHODS**: The study included 11 patients who had undergone orthognathic surgery at least six months previously, had received speech therapy and had no peri- or post-operative complications or neurological diseases. The aspect and postural condition of the structures of the stomatognathic system were observed, of which only the position of the tongue and the aspect of the hard palate were within the normal range, and the mobility of the structures was assessed. All were below the normal range. A glass of water, a small portion of hazelnut and cocoa cream (Nutella®) and a filled biscuit were offered to assess stomatognathic functions. The behaviour of the lips and tongue during swallowing and the type of chewing were slightly below the normal range. **CONCLUSION**: Based on the results, it was possible to conclude that patients undergoing orthognathic surgery and speech therapy had orofacial myofunctional aspects close to the normal range.

Keywords: stomatognathic system, orthognathic surgery, orofacial motricity, dentofacial deformities.

SUMMARY

CHAPTER 1

1. INTRODUCTION

The stomatognathic system identifies a set of oral structures that perform common functions, with the mandible being a constant feature. It is made up of bone tissue, teeth, muscles, nerves and vessels that are related in a complex way, despite having their own biology and functional structure, adapted to specific functions (DOUGLAS, C. R. apud PEREIRA et al, 2005).

The harmonious relationship between the components of this system favours adequate growth and development of the facial bone bases (PEREIRA etal, 2005).

Changes in the dynamics of this system interfere with craniofacial growth in such a way as to jeopardise the functions of breathing, chewing, swallowing and speech (KIYAK, McNEILL and WEST, 1985).

Deformities can occur in the vertical, transverse and horizontal directions. The facial pattern influences the findings regarding stomatognathic functions in individuals with skeletal Class III malocclusion, with the dolichocephalic type contributing to alterations in habitual lip posture, as well as breathing and speech functions, while the mesocephalic type influences the swallowing characteristics of individuals with skeletal Class III malocclusion (PEREIRA et al, 2005).

The literature suggests that there is no difference in maximum isometric bite force between the different patterns of dentofacial deformities (class II and class III), however, the values for these two groups were lower than normal individuals, showing that deformity, regardless of its pattern, affects this bite force (TRAWITZKI et al, 2008).

Orthodontic treatment associated with orthognathic surgery has brought solutions to these patients, with reports of: improved facial aesthetics, improved masticatory functions, improved phonetic functions and reduced joint and myofacial pain (AMBRIZZI et al, 2007).

The benefits may be even greater with interdisciplinary treatment. Trawitzki et al. (2010) reported that the electromyographic activity of the masseter muscle improved in a patient with class III dentofacial deformity over a three-year period after treatment with an interdisciplinary team, reaching values close to those of normal individuals. In the interdisciplinary treatment, the patient is periodically monitored by professionals from different areas of the same service, who discuss the case as a team, resulting in better integration between professionals and patients.

The speech therapist is the professional qualified to carry out orofacial myofunctional therapy in order to restore the balance of stomatognathic functions.

Post-surgical changes tend to stabilise over time, as the soft tissues readapt to the new spaces. During the speech therapy process, it is noted that many of them manage to actually modify their functions and others only incorporate them, which is considered satisfactory. However, in some cases, speech, chewing and swallowing are not very satisfactory, even a year after surgery (MARCHESAN and BIANCHINI, 1999).

1.1. OBJECTIVES

GENERAL OBJECTIVE

Defining orofacial myofunctional aspects in patients who have undergone orthognathic surgery and speech therapy in the post operative period.

SPECIFIC OBJECTIVES

To assess the appearance and postural condition, mobility and functions of the stomatognathic system, with emphasis on the oral phase of swallowing.

CHAPTER 2

2. CASUISTRY AND METHODS

2.1. ETHICAL CONSIDERATIONS

This study was carried out with the written consent of each participant, expressed in specific terms for the different procedures, after they had been duly informed. The research was approved by the Research Ethics Committee of the São José do Rio Preto Medical School.

2.2. TYPE OF STUDY

The research has a quantitative approach in which the systematic collection of information will provide numerical information and enable the researcher to systematically evaluate the subject. It is a cross-sectional study, allowing the evaluation of data existing at the time of collection; it is also descriptive with the description of the average of the variables studied.

2.3. PLACE OF STUDY

The research was carried out at the Otorhinolaryngology, Orthodontics and Speech and Hearing Therapy department of the Specialities Outpatient Clinic at the Hospital de Base in São José do Rio Preto/SP.

2.4. CHARACTERISATION OF THE SAMPLE

Data was collected from patients undergoing orthognathic surgery at this service. Participants were recruited by telephone call and on their return to the outpatient clinic after being seen by the specialist, and no influencing actions were allowed. Those who voluntarily agreed to take part were included in the study by signing an informed consent form.

2.5. INCLUSION AND EXCLUSION CRITERIA

The research subjects were obtained after establishing the criteria described below.

- Individuals who consented to take part in the study;
- Who underwent orthognathic surgery for both maxillary advancement and mandibular retraction at least six months and no more than ten years ago;
- Who underwent speech therapy;
- Who had no complications in the peri- and post-operative period;
- Who do not have glucose intolerance;

- Who have no history of stroke or neurological disease.

These criteria were certified by the researcher prior to data collection. In line with the study's methodological requirements, the employees were invited to undergo an orofacial myofunctional assessment using the Orofacial Myofunctional Assessment with Scores (AMIOFE) protocol proposed by Felício and Ferreira (2008). The items were assessed using scores according to their characteristics, with the maximum and minimum scores varying from item to item.

2.6. METHODOLOGICAL PROCEDURES

The orofacial myofunctional assessment took place with the patient seated in a comfortable chair, where observation began of the postural condition of the lips and jaw and the appearance of the cheeks, tongue, hard palate and facial symmetry.

The mobility of the lips, tongue, mandible and cheeks was also assessed, based on the verbal command and model given by the assessor to perform the movements of elevation, lowering, lateralisation, protrusion and retraction of these structures.

The participant was then asked to swallow water from a disposable cup and a small amount of Nutella® (hazelnut cream with milk and cocoa) deposited on the anterior portion of the tongue, in order to help the researcher visualise the point to be touched by the tongue during the oral phase of swallowing. In normal individuals, the tip of the tongue rests against the edges of the maxillary alveolus or the upper incisors. However, the muscular alterations present in individuals undergoing orthognathic surgery can lead to the installation of adapted swallowing, which is often difficult to diagnose due to the limitations of visualisation within the oral cavity during swallowing.

In the swallowing function, in addition to tongue behaviour, lip and facial muscle behaviour was observed, as well as checking for food escapes and compensatory head movements.

In individuals who have undergone orthognathic surgery, the orbicularis oris muscle may be under-functioning due to malocclusion, which can cause excessive contraction of the mentonian musculature, as a form of compensation, and the escape of food when the lip seal is absent or inefficient.

Compensatory head movements are related to inefficient propulsion of the food bolus. This is due to the altered tongue tone found in individuals with malocclusion.

Swallowing efficiency was another item assessed. The need

to perform multiple swallows may suggest that the structures of the stomatognathic system are not performing their function satisfactorily.

The chewing function was assessed by offering a chocolate-flavoured Bono® brand biscuit. The type of chewing and the presence of altered behaviours/signs were observed.

Breathing function was assessed by the assessor observing the patient at rest.

The Orofacial Myofunctional Assessment Protocol with Scores, proposed by Felício and Ferreira (2008), was used for the assessment, and the entire procedure was filmed using a Sony®Cyber-Shot digital camera, 16.2 mega pixels.

CHAPTER 3

3. RESULTS

Eleven patients took part in the study, 6 women and 5 men, all of whom had undergone maxillary advancement surgery. The results were presented in descriptive and illustrative form using tables.

3.1. Results of postural aspects and conditions

The postural aspects and conditions of the facial structures were observed with the patient sitting in a comfortable chair at the start of the orofacial myofunctional assessment. **Table 1** shows the values found for these parameters.

Table 1- Description of the mean postural condition of the lips and jaw, appearance of the cheeks, facial symmetry, position of the tongue and appearance of the hard palate obtained by the patients and the maximum and minimum scores.

Postural appearance and condition	)tida (scores)	(scores)

Postural condition of the lips	2,8	2-3
Postural condition of the mandible	2,7	2-3
Appearance of the cheeks	2,1	1-3
Facial symmetry	2,2	1-3
Tongue position	3	3
Appearance of the hard palate	2,9	2-3

As for the postural condition of the lips and jaw, the mean scores of 2.8 and 2.7 were below the normal range of 3 scores. However, the difference was minimal, with only 0.2 and 0.3 scores.

The mean scores for cheek appearance and facial symmetry were 2.1, also below the normal range of 3 scores.

The mean tongue position score was 2.9, with a difference of just 0.1 below the normal range. The hard palate aspect achieved the maximum score of 3.

3.2. Mobility

The mobility of the lips, tongue, mandible and cheeks was assessed using the verbal command and model given by the assessor to perform the movements of elevation, lowering, lateralisation, protrusion and retraction of these structures. **Table 2** shows the values found for each structure.

Table 2- Description of the average lip, tongue, jaw and cheek movements obtained by the patients and the maximum and minimum scores.

Mobility	score (scores)	maximum score and ia (scores)
Lip movements	10,8	8-12
Tongue movements	16	13-18
Jaw movements	13,8	10-15
Cheek movements	11,3	9-12

All the averages obtained for the mobility of each structure were below normal, with 10.8 scores for lip movements, 16 scores for tongue movements, 13.8 scores for jaw movements and 11.3 scores for cheek movements, which had a normal range of 12, 18, 15 and 12 scores, respectively.

3.3. Functions

The functions of breathing at rest, swallowing (oral phase) and chewing were assessed.

To assess swallowing function, the participant was asked to swallow water from a disposable cup and a small amount of Nutella® (hazelnut cream with milk and cocoa) deposited on the anterior portion of the tongue, in order to observe the behaviour of the lips, tongue, other behaviours and signs of alteration and the efficiency of swallowing.

The chewing function was assessed by offering a chocolate-flavoured Bono® brand biscuit. The type of chewing and the presence of altered behaviours/signs were observed. **Table 3** shows the values found for each item observed.

Table 3- Description of the mean scores for breathing, swallowing (lip and tongue behaviour, other behaviours and signs of alteration and swallowing efficiency), chewing (chewing type and other behaviours and signs of alteration) obtained by the patients and the lowest and highest scores possible.

Functions	**day obtained ^scores)**	**maximum score and ia (scores)**
Breathing	3	3
Swallowing - lip behaviour	2,5	2-3
Swallowing - tongue behaviour	2,7	2-3
Swallowing - other behaviours and signs of change	2,3	1-3
Swallowing efficiency	2,8	1-3
Chewing - masticatory type	2,9	2-4
Chewing - other behaviours and signs of change	2,7	2-3

Only the breathing function had a maximum mean, which was within normal standards.

The other items had averages below expectations. However, it is worth noting that the items: swallowing - tongue behaviour; swallowing efficiency; chewing - chewing type; and chewing - other behaviours and signs of alteration, were below the normal range, with scores of 2.7; 2.8; 2.9; and 2.7, with a difference of only 0.3- 0.1 below the normal range.

CHAPTER 4

4. DISCUSSION

The study by Oland, Jensen and Meisen (2010) indicated that orthognathic surgery improves stomatognathic functions in most cases, and that this improvement was also reported by patients at the end of treatment. However, the author emphasises that in none of the cases did the functions reach the level of the control group.

In their clinical practice, Marchesan and Bianchini (1999) observed cases in which even after repositioning the bone bases, the expected muscle changes were not achieved. In these circumstances, speech therapy work consists fundamentally of functional re-education, seeking to direct the musculature through the use of stomatognathic functions within the individual's new possibilities.

In our study, in general terms, we observed that although the difference was small, the muscles and functions of chewing and swallowing were also below normal standards, showing adaptations of the structures of the stomatognathic system to perform their functions. This confirms the findings of this study and the data from the references cited in it. Nakata et al. (2007) showed that the masticatory muscles in patients with mandibular prognathism can adapt to the new environment created by surgical correction of the dentofacial structure, but that the muscles remain at low levels compared to normal individuals.

Adaptive patterns can set in due to the sudden change in the structures of the stomatognathic system, so a new proprioceptive scheme must be acquired so that the soft tissue structures can perform their functions satisfactorily (MARCHESAN and BIANCHINI, 1999).

Trawitzki et al. (2010) studied the EMG activity of the masseter muscle in patients who had undergone orthognathic surgery three years previously and found values close to those of normal individuals.

Marchesan and Bianchini (1999) reported that structures undergo changes over time after surgery, both slow and delayed.

However, perhaps we could have found more satisfactory results in our study if our group of participants had been made up of individuals who had undergone orthognathic surgery more recently.

CHAPTER 5

5. CONCLUSION

The results show that the orofacial myofunctional aspects of patients undergoing orthognathic surgery and speech therapy are close to normal.

CHAPTER 6

6 BIBLIOGRAPHICAL REFERENCES

AMBRIZZI, D. R.; FRANZI, S.A.; PEREIRA-FILHO, V. A.; GABRIELLI, M. A. C.; GIMENEZ, C.M.M.M.; BERTOZ, F.A. Evaluation of aesthetic-functional complaints in patients with dentofacial deformities. Rev. Dental Press Ortodontia e Ortopedia Facial, V. 12, n. 5, p. 63-70, Sep/Oct, 2007.

DOUGLAS, C. R. Physiologia geral do sistema estomatognático.In: Tratado de fisiologia aplicada a fonoaudiologia apud PEREIRA, A.C.; JORGE, T.M.; JÚNIOR, P.D.R.; BERRETIN-FELIX, G. Características das funções orais de indivíduos com má occlusão Classe III e diferentes tipos. Rev. Dental Press Ortodontia e Ortopedia Facial, v. 10, n. 6, p. 111-119, nov./dez, 2005.

FELÍCIO C.M.; FERREIRA, C. L. Protocol of orofacial myofunctional evaluation with scores. International Journal of Paediatric Otorhinolaryngology. Elsevier, v. 72, p. 367-375, 2008.

KIYAK, H. A.; McNEILL, R. W.; WEST, R. A. The emotional impact of orthognathic surgery and conventional Orthodonthics.Am. J. Orthod., St. Louis, v. 88, p. 224-234, 1985.

MARCHESAN, I.Q.; BIANCHINI, E.M.G. Speech and hearing therapy and orthognathic surgery. In: Araújo MCA. Orthognathic surgery. São Paulo, 1999.

NAKATA, Y.; UEDA, H.M.; KATO, M.; TABE, H.; SHIKATA-WAKISAKA, N.; MATSUMOTO, E.; KOH, M.; TANAKA, E.; TANNE, K. Changes in Stomatognathic Function Induced by Orthognathic Surgery in Patients With

Mandibular Prognathism. Journal of Oral and Maxillofacial Surgery, v. 65:444451,2007.

OLAND, J.; JENSEN, J.; MELSEN,B. Factors of Importance for the Functional

Outcome in Orthognathic Surgery Patients: A Prospective Study of 118 Patients. Journal of Oral and Maxillofacial Surgery, v. 68:2221-2231, 2010.

PEREIRA, A.C.; JORGE, T.M.; JÚNIOR, P.D.R.; BERRETIN-FELIX, G. Characteristics of the oral functions of individuals with Class III malocclusion and different types. Rev. Dental Press Ortodontia e Ortopedia Facial, v. 10, n. 6, p. 111-119, nov./dez, 2005.

TRAWITZKI, L.V.V. ; SILVA, J.B.; REGALO, S.C.H.; MELO-FILHO,

F.V. Effect of class II and class III dentofacial deformities under orthodontic treatment on maximal isometric bite force. Archives of oral biology, v. 56, p. 972-976, 2008.

TRAWITZKI, L.V.V.; DANTAS, R.O.; MELLO-FILHO, F.V.; MARQUES JR, W. Masticatory muscle function three years after surgical correction of class III dentofacial deformity. Int Journal of Oral and Maxillofacial Surgery, v. 39:853-6, 2010.

CHAPTER 7

ANNEX 1

INFORMED CONSENT FORM

Study title: "Orofacial myofunctional profile of patients undergoing

orthognathic surgery

surgery"

Name of participant: ______________________________

Address:

____

____

Telephone: (_____) ____ -

You are being invited to take part in a scientific study that could increase your knowledge of the muscles of the mouth and face and their functions, such as chewing, swallowing and breathing. These aspects may be altered even after the surgery you have undergone. If so, we will provide you with speech therapy to adjust. This study will be carried out to improve knowledge on this subject and even provide data so that we can improve the treatment of people who undergo the same procedure.

WHAT IS THE STUDY ABOUT?

To feed ourselves, we use a set of oral structures, such as bones, teeth, muscles, nerves and blood vessels, which together perform the functions of breathing, swallowing and chewing.

Changes in these functions interfere with orthodontic treatment associated with orthognathic surgery, which aims to improve facial aesthetics, improve masticatory functions and reduce pain in the joints and muscles of the face.

However, in some cases, chewing and swallowing are unsatisfactory, even a year after surgery.

The speech therapist is the professional qualified to restore the muscles of the face and balance the functions of breathing, swallowing and chewing.

The aim of this study is to see if, even after orthognathic surgery and speech therapy, the muscles and functions of breathing, swallowing and chewing are close to normal.

HOW WILL THE STUDY BE CARRIED OUT?

Participants in the study will be invited by telephone. No influencing actions of any kind will be allowed.

The study will be carried out as follows:

a) the researcher will observe the structures of the participant's face;

b) you will be asked to make movements with your lips, such as: making a beak, moving the beak from side to side, and smiling;

c) movements with the tongue, such as: sticking it out of the mouth, moving it to the right, left, up, down and into the mouth;

d) jaw movements: opening the mouth, closing the mouth, moving the jaw from side to side and forwards;

e) cheek movements: filling the cheeks with air, moving the air from one side to the other and emptying them completely;

f) ingesting a glass of water, a small amount of Nutella® chocolate and a chocolate-flavoured Bono® biscuit to see how the participant chews and swallows.

The entire procedure will be recorded by a digital camera.

ARE THESE PROCEDURES UNCOMFORTABLE OR RISKY?

The procedures will not involve any health risks and/or

discomfort for the participant.

WHAT HAPPENS TO THOSE WHO DON'T TAKE PART IN THE STUDY?

Nothing will happen to you if you don't want to take part in this study.

Your refusal to take part in this research will also be accepted, as will your withdrawal at any time, without any prejudice to the continuity of any treatment at this institution, penalty or any kind of damage to your person. Your identity will be kept completely confidential and at any time you can withdraw your data from being used in this research.

You will not incur any expenses for taking part in the research throughout the duration of the study. There will also be no financial rewards related to your participation.

Finally, if you feel you have been harmed, you have the right to request compensation, in accordance with current legislation, although no compensation is provided for at . You will be fully supervised and free to ask questions and clarify your doubts at any stage of this study. If you have any questions or problems with the research, you can contact the researcher in charge, Patricia Moraes Pereira, by e-mail atpatriciapereira18@hotmail.com or by telephone: (17) 3201-5000, ext. 1205 - speech therapy department of the

Specialities Outpatient Clinic of the Hospital de Base de São José do Rio Preto - SP.

Priscila Piassi Carboni

Researcher in Charge

Isabel Cristina Figueiredo

Advisor

Research Participant or Responsible Person

RG: ______________________

ANNEX 2

AMIOFE Protocol

DN:

User:

Current Age:

Evaluation date:

Appearance and Postural Condition/Position

Postural Condition of the Lips		**Scores**
Sealed	They fulfil their function normally	(3)
Sealed with Voltage	They fulfil their function, but with excessive contraction of the lips and Mm. Mentual	(2)
Between the doors	Mild dysfunction	(2)
Fully open	Severe dysfunction	(1)
Subject result evaluated		

Postural Condition of the Jaw		Scores
Normal postural condition	Maintains EFL	(3)
Teeth in occlusion or edge contact	Tightening	(2)
Lowered (lips parted)	Mild dysfunction	(2)
Down (mouth open)	Severe dysfunction	(1)
Appearance of the cheeks		**Scores**
	Normal	(3)
Asymmetry	Lightweight	(2)
	Severe	(1)
Flaccid	Severe	(1)
Evaluated subject's result		
Facial symmetry		**Scores**
Symmetry between right and left sides	Normal	(3)
Asymmetry	Lightweight	(2)

	Severe		(1)
Enlarged side	Law	Left	
Evaluated subject's result			
Tongue position			**Scores**
Contained in the oral cavity	Normal		(3)
Interposed with the dental arches	Adaptation or dysfunction		(2)
	Overproduced		(1)
Evaluated subject's result			
Appearance of the Hard Palate			**Scores**
	Normal		(3)
Narrow width	Lightweight		(2)
	Severo		(1)
Evaluated subject's result			

Mobility

PERFORMANCE	LIP MOVEMENTS				
	Protrusion	Shrinkage	Laterality D	Laterality E	Scores
Normal	(3)	(3)	(3)	(3)	
Skill Insufficient tremor	(2)	(2)	(2)	(2)	
No skill	(1)	(1)	(1)	(1)	
Not realised	(1)	(1)	(1)	(1)	
				Sum	

Performance	TONGUE MOVEMENTS						
	Protrude	Retract	Side D	Side E	Elevate	Lower	Scores
Normal	(3)	(3)	(3)	(3)	(3)	(3)	
Insufficient ability tremor	(2)	(2)	(2)	(2)	(2)	(2)	
No skill	(1)	(1)	(1)	(1)	(1)	(1)	

Not realised	(1)	(1)	(1)	(1)	(1)	(1)	
					Sum		

PERFORMANCE	JAW MOVEMENTS					
	Lower	Elevate	Side D	Side E	Protrude	**Scores**
Normal	(3)	(3)	(3)	(3)	(3)	
Insufficient skill deviation	(2)	(2)	(2)	(2)	(2)	
No skill	(1)	(1)	(1)	(1)	(1)	
Not realised	(1)	(1)	(1)	(1) Sum	(1)	

PERFORMANCE	CHEEK MOVEMENTS				
	Inflate	Smother	Retract	Lateralising the air	**Scores**
Normal	(3)	(3)	(3)	(3)	

Insufficient skill deviation	(2)	(2)	(2)	(2)	
No skill	(0)	(0)	(0)	(0)	
Not realised	(0)	(0)	(0)	(0)	
				Sum	

FUNCTIONS

Breathing		**Scores**
Nasal breathing	Normal	(3)
Oronasal breathing	Lightweight	(2)
	Severe	(1)
Evaluated subject's result		

Swallowing: Lip behaviour		Scores
Seals the Oral Cavity	Without seeming to make an effort	(3)
They seal the oral	Lightweight	(2)

cavity, but contract more than normal	Severe	(1)
the Oral Cavity	Doesn't fulfil its function	(0)
Evaluated subject's result		

Swallowing: Tongue behaviour		Scores
Contained in the oral cavity	Normal	(3)
Interposed with the dental arches	Adaptation or dysfunction	(2)
	Overproduced	(1)
Evaluated subject's result		

Swallowing: Other behaviours and signs of change		
		Scores
Head movement	Absent	(1)
	Present	(0)

Muscle Tension	Absent	(1)
	Present	(0)
Escape of food	Absent	(1)
	Present	(0)
Evaluated subject's result		

Swallowing Efficiency Complementary Item -	**Scores**
Solid cake	
Does not repeat swallowing the same cake	(3)
A repeat	(2)
Multiple swallows	(1)
Liquid Cake	
Does not repeat swallowing the same cake	(3)
A repeat	(2)
Multiple swallows	(1)

Results

Total Swallowing Result	

Chewing		Scores
Bilateral	Alternating	(4)
	Simultaneous (vertical)	(3)
Unilateral	Preferential (66%)	(2)
	Chronicle	(1)
Anterior (Frontal)		(1)

Does not fulfil the function	No grinding	(1)
Evaluated subject's result		

Other behaviours and signs of change		Scores
Movement of the head or other parts of the body	Absent	(1)
	Present	(0)
Altered posture	Absent	(1)
	Present	(0)
Escape of food	Absent	(1)
	Present	(0)
Evaluated subject's		

result	
Total Chewing Result	
Time taken to eat the food =	
Food used =	

Considerations of the examiner:
Examiner/CRFa:

Source: FELÍCIO C.M.; FERREIRA, C. L. Protocol of orofacial myofunctional evaluation with scores. International Journal of Paediatric Otorhinolaryngology. Elsevier, v. 72, p. 367375, 2008.

Druck:
CPI Druckdienstleistungen GmbH
im Auftrag der
Kolibri 360 GmbH
Ferdinand-Jühlke-Str. 7
99095 Erfurt

Kolibri 360 GmbH
Ferdinand-Jühlke-Straße 7
99095 Erfurt, Deutschland
produktsicherheit@kolibri360.de